KEG

WOMEN

Solution to Urinary Incontinence, Better Sex Life and Strengthen Pelvic Floor Muscles

BY

Patrick Elizabeth

Table of Contents

Chapter 1

Kegel Exercise

Kegel exercise is a very important exercise for women because it enables us to develop a healthy pelvic floor muscles. The Kegel practices have been popular over the couple of years due to is great benefit.

Healthy pelvic floor muscles are something that any lady should go for in her life. Tragically, these muscles are the least exercise and the most disregarded by generally ladies. Which prompts expanded danger of urinary, fecal and stress incontinence for a great deal of ladies all around the globe.

Kegel practices are exceptionally structured activities that plan to fortify your pelvic floor muscles, which are the muscles that hold your rectum, bladder, uterus and small digestive tract. A few elements can influence the state of your pelvic floor muscles, for example, pregnancy, conceiving an offspring and medical surgery, can present you to high dangers of urinary, stress and fecal incontinence.

Kegel practices are the ideal method to decrease these dangers for yourself, these activities are likewise the absolute most economical and regular treatment of urinary, stress and fecal incontinence.

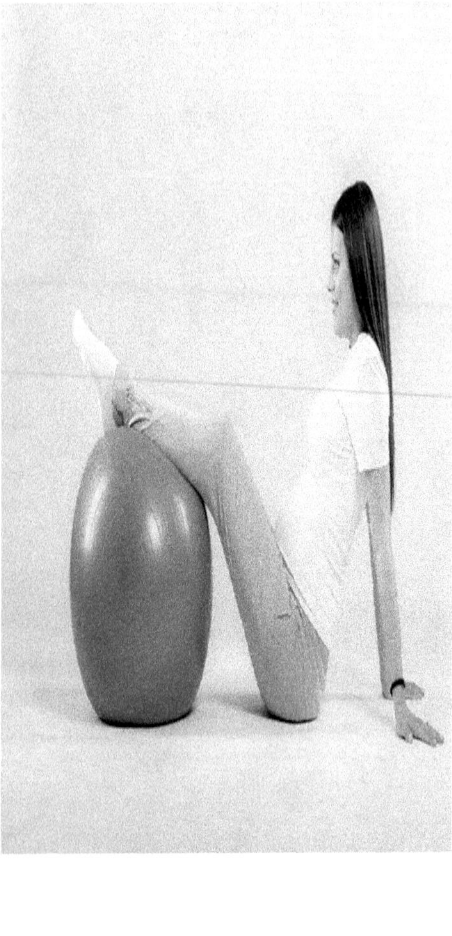

Chapter 2

Benefit Of Kegel Exercise

One of the objective of kegel practice is to reinforce the pelvic floor muscles, there are alot of advantage of kegel practice for ladies they are

1. Kegel controls urinary incontinence

2. Kegel help to lessen pelvic organ prolapsed (POP)

3. It helps in Recovery After birth

4. It help pelvic floor amid menopause

5. Great Sex

Kegel controls urinary incontinence

The term incontinence alludes to automatic or incidental loss of either pee (urinary incontinence) from the bladder. While this issue can cause extensive humiliation, it is entirely normal and in excess of 13 million Americans are living with urinary incontinence. As per inquire about from the National Association for Continence, 20% of people age 40 or over will experience the ill effects of an overactive bladder with recurrence and desperation side effects, and some may spill pee before they achieve the restroom. While looking at the number of inhabitants in more established grown-ups who live in nursing homes, over half of occupants experience the ill effects of urinary incontinence.

Roughly 1 out of 20 individuals experience issues controlling their urine, and this issue will turn out to be increasingly with age

Kegel practices are the most characteristic and powerful approach to control urinary incontinence (UI). Regardless of your age, people alike who experience the ill effects of this issue can profit by taking part in Kegel practices all the time. The individuals who experience the ill effects of urinary incontinence ordinarily have weak pelvic floor muscles. Kegel practices strengthen this muscles which help in the condition of urinary incontinence.

You would profit from Kegel practices greatly if you are experiencing any of this:

- A sudden, compelling impulse to urinate before losing a huge of measure of pee
- Spilling when hacking, chuckling or sniffling
- Stool spillage

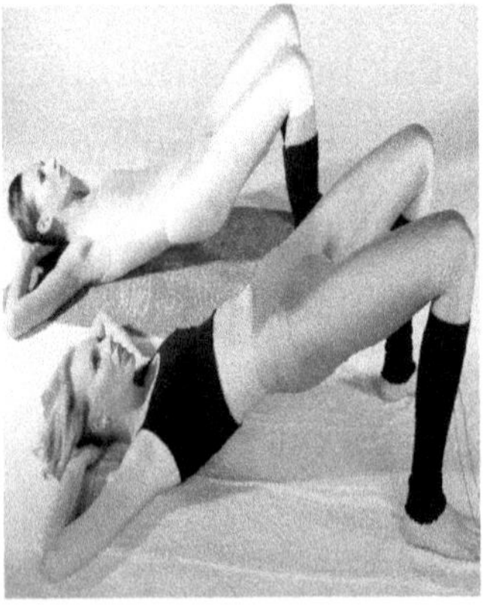

Chapter 3

Kegel help to lessen pelvic organ prolapsed (POP)

Pelvic organ prolapse is a condition in which at least one of the pelvic organs presses into the walls of vagina. This generally happens after the pelvic floor muscles have been weakened, for example, after pregnancy and labor.

Ladies may likewise have POP from continous heavy lifting, they can also develop it as a result of obesity or cough. Pelvic organ prolapse isn't dangerous, however it can cause torment, dread, and issues with the bladder. It can likewise prompt by and large diminished satisfaction throughout everyday life.

Pelvic organ prolapse is a condition described by an impression of pressure in the vagina. Regularly, these can be felt in different degrees by setting a finger into the vaginal.

They can likewise be seen utilizing a hand-held mirror to watch the vaginal opening. It might feel as if the pelvic organs have turned out to be heavy, or just as they are dropping out of the body. The pressure might be more terrible at night or after exercise or physical activities.

It isn't phenomenal to encounter odd spilling after pee, particularly when standing up from the toilet.

POP is brought about by tearing and debilitating of the pelvic floor muscles themselves or the ligaments suspending the organs. It is evaluated that half of ladies who have had a baby will encounter prolapse to some degree.

Age likewise is a factor in growing POP for half of ladies who are 50 years old and older.

Pushing that happen during labour, tearing of pelvic floor during child birth and delivery a bigger baby are generally factors that can prompt prolapse.

Ladies who are on second or more births are at higher hazard for POP to happen. Ladies who have experienced C-Section can likewise encounter POP now and again. Heavy lifting and sit ups ought to be maintained a strategic distance from, as this can prompt intensifying of the prolapse.

The incredible news is that Kegels can fortify the pelvic floor muscles for better help of the pelvic organs and decrease of prolapse. Low dimensions of prolapse can be totally relieved, and moderate dimensions of prolapse can be diminished to the point where they don't meddle with everyday life exercises.

Chapter4

It helps in Recovery after birth

The landing of an infant is the most awesome involvement in a lady's life; be that as it may, conceiving an offspring can likewise inflict significant damage on her body. While you need to ensure that things run easily for your new conceived, you will likewise need to guarantee their prosperity and wellbeing. You should rest soundly, eat well and deal with your weight. Other than managing these, you will likewise need to strengthen your pelvic floor muscles.

Delivery leads to the weakening of the pelvic floor muscles. The most ideal approach to fortify pelvic muscles is with the Kegel practices.

Kegel practices are gainful when you're pregnant and keep on offering benefits after the delivering of your baby.

Kegel practices after labor are required for recuperating the debilitated, stressed or harmed pelvic muscles from pushing the child through the vaginal. Vaginal muscles, uterus and cervix may get torn during delivery. These muscles should be mended and fortified to keep away from medical problems in the long haul. Kegels will expand the blood dissemination to these regions and help the healing.

Regardless of whether you have the child through cesarean or normal process, you will have issues with bladder control. Urinary spillage issues are regular after labor. An extending uterus can put a great deal of weight on your pelvic floor muscles and debilitate them. This can be humiliating in broad daylight particularly when you laugh, cough or sneeze. Kegel practice afterbirth fortifies pelvic floor muscles and helps you with bladder control.

Chapter 5

It help pelvic floor amid menopause

Amid the time paving the way to menopause, frequently call perimenopause, you see changes in your body, including menstrual cycle, inconvenience sleeping and more. Likewise, you may see an adjustment in your wellbeing. Regardless of what side effect you're battling with amid this confused time, realize that arrangements and adapting techniques exist that can help, and always ensure to consult your doctor during this time.

Amid perimenopause, decreasing estrogen levels can make your vaginal tissues lose oil and flexibility.

Along these lines, you may see the some changes:

1. Urinary Incontinence.

2. Dyspareunia: Sexual activities become painful.

3. Pelvic Organ Prolapse

These personal issues may huge affect your life, the response to enhancing or avoiding them is some of the time as straightforward as including a couple of minutes of no-sweat exercise to your day by day schedule.

Kegel practicing will be of great help during your whole life. Building your pelvic floor muscles will assist you with having better bladder control.

Chapter 6

Kegel improves Sex Life

With regards to sex, Kegel practices make the vagina feel more tightly and may help enhance the power of the climax. The pelvic floor muscles are indispensable with regards to climax.

They are in charge of the pleasurable constrictions felt in the privates when a climax happens. At the point when the pelvic floor muscles are sound, climaxes are progressively intense and last more. Ladies who experience issues accomplishing climax might encounter frail pelvic floor muscles.

Strengthening pelvic floor leads to increase blood flow, improve ability to climax, increase sexual arousal as well as lubrication.

Moreover, a solid pelvic floor enables ladies to grasp their men during sexual intercourse, which is pleasurable for the man too.

Adaptable pelvic floor muscles make vaginal penetration easy. Ladies who experience difficult entrance should see a pelvic physical specialist as they might encounter vaginismus, which is the frequently painful automatic contraction of vaginal.

Vaginismus it is treatable, and kegel can prompt pleasurable intercourse without pelvic torment.

Chapter 7

How to Perform Kegel Exercise

Kegel practices are carried out by squeezing the muscles in the pelvic floor and holding it. To start you have to:

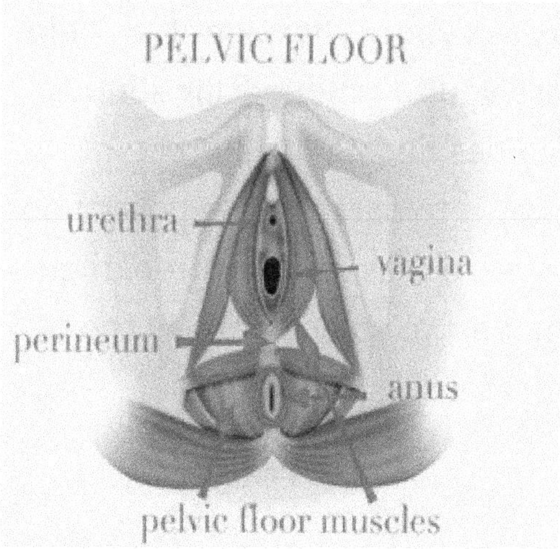

Locate the correct muscles.

One approach to locate the correct muscle is by endeavoring to stop the stream of pee whenever you go to the bathroom. The muscle you use to control the flow of urine is the pelvic floor muscle, which is the muscle needed for Kegel practise. Another approach to test is to put your finger into your vagina and attempt to squeeze it. Try not to be hesitant to approach your gynecologist for help in case you're experiencing serious difficulties finding the correct muscle. The key is to detect these pelvic floor muscles so that you can strengthen them. Ensure you're working the correct muscle.

Start your kegel Slowly

Begin moderate and develop. In case you're new to Kegel work out, begin moderate. Squeeze your pelvic muscle and hold for three to five seconds and then relax. Endeavor to repeat 5 to 12 times. As this activity gets easier, you can hold for longer timeframes and ensure to repeat for a couple of time.

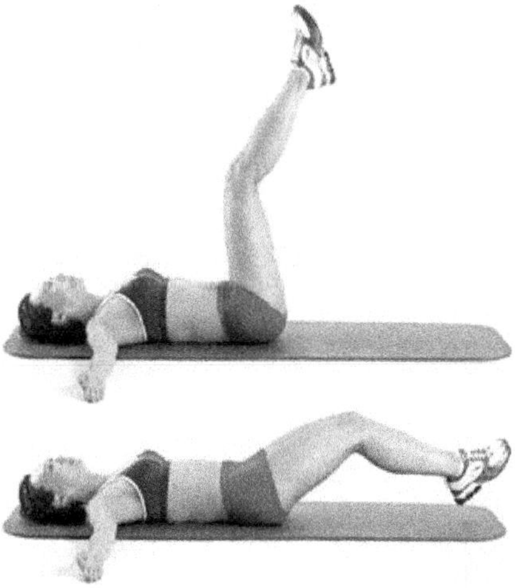

Ensure to do Kegel Regularly

Once you are used to kegel you can always do them any time at your own comfort. You can also form a routine on how you will be doing it.

Speak with your gynecologist in the event that despite everything you aren't sure you've discovered the correct muscles. They may prescribe utilizing an object called a vaginal cone. You embed a vaginal cone into the vagina and after that utilization your pelvic floor muscles to keep it set up.

Biofeedback can likewise be exceptionally valuable in identifying your pelvic floor muscles. In this method, a specialist will embed a probe into your vagina. You'll be approached to attempt to complete a Kegel. It will indicate on a screen whether you gotten the right muscles and to what extent you could hold the contraction.

THE END

CPSIA information can be obtained
at www.ICGtesting.com
Printed in the USA
LVHW081708180721
693019LV00021B/1234

9 781797 655338